Amino Acids

A Nutritional Guide

Use for:
- Mental Clarity (with SAF® chain work)
- Correcting Deficiencies
- Finding Synergists

Kathy M. Scogna

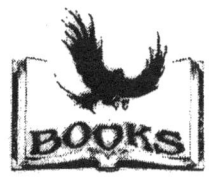

Amino Acids—A Nutritional Guide
by Kathy M. Scogna

For mental clarity with SAF® chain work; for discovering deficiencies and synergists

Copyright © 1983, 2014
By Kathy M. Scogna
All Rights Reserved

No part of this book may be reproduced or transmitted in any form or by any means, electronic or mechanical including photocopying, recording, or by any information storage retrieval system without permission of the copyright owner.

Published in the USA by: Life Energy Publications
www.LifeEnergyResearch.com

SAF® is a registered trademark and signifies that this is part of the collective work and research of Joseph R. Scogna, Jr.

Amino Acids: A Nutritional Guide
Includes illustrations, index

    1. Amino acids   2. Self help   3. Self awareness
    4. SAF® method   5. SAF Online

    I. Kathy M. Scogna, author   II. Title

ISBN: 13: 978-1505690231
ISBN: 10: 1505690234

Amino Acids
A Nutritional Guide

For mental clarity with SAF® chain work;
for discovering deficiencies and synergists

Note to the Reader: there is no intent to diagnose or treat any disease with the information in this book. If disease or ill health is present, a qualified practitioner should be consulted.

The information is presented here for dual educational purposes: for SAF® practitioners to use for a mental assist in charity of images, and for practitioners interested in symptomatic patterns and physical deficiencies.

Table of Contents

Introduction 1
Use for Mental Assist & to Correct a Deficiency 3
Alanine 5
Arginine 7
Aspartic acid 9
Asparagine 11
Cysteine and Cystine 12
Glutamic acid 14
Glutamine 16
Glycine 18
Histidine 20
Hydroxyproline 22
Isoleucine 24
Leucine 26
Lysine 27
Methionine 29
Phenylalanine 31
Proline 33
Serine 35
Threonine 37
Tryptophan 39
Tyrosine 41
Valine 43
Essential Amino Acids List 45
References 45
Index 46

INTRODUCTION

Protoplasm is the living material, the energy, of all cells in plants and animals. It is a fluid, consisting of 75-90% water with the remaining solids being mostly protein with fatty substances, carbohydrates, organic and inorganic compounds. Innumerable reactions and energy transfers occur within protoplasm, making it alive, more than merely an assortment of proteins and other material. Studies continue in an attempt to discover still more about protoplasm, the very essence of life itself.

The protein molecules found within protoplasm are thousands of times larger than water molecules. When food is digested, the proteins in it are broken down into amino acids, the structural units or building blocks of which proteins are composed. These amino acids, containing carbon, hydrogen, oxygen, nitrogen and sometimes sulfur, are linked together in long chains of perhaps 200-300 or more to form the protein molecule. The kind of protein formed is dependent upon the number, kind and arrangement of these amino acid formulas.

$$H_2N-\underset{\underset{H}{|}}{\overset{\overset{R}{|}}{C}}-C\underset{OH}{\overset{O}{\diagup\!\!\!\diagdown}}$$

General formula of an amino acid

Amino acids are essential to plant and animal life. Twenty-two amino acids are found in animals; over 100 less common ones in plants. Green plants can synthesize all their amino acids; animals normally have to obtain their supply directly from plants or indirectly by eating other animals which have eaten plants. The amino acids needed by animals, and this includes man, can be divided into the essential and non-essential. Here, essential means that animals do not construct these from materials in the body but rather these amino acids must be supplied, preformed and derived originally from protein food. The non-essential amino acids are also needed but they can be constructed within the body chiefly in the liver by the transformation of one amino acid to another. Amino acids compete with one another. Man, therefore, needs an adequate total number of amino acids plus an ample supply of the essential amino acids.

Most animal protein foods, such as eggs, milk, and meat contain all of the essential amino acids and are therefore classified as high quality proteins. Gelatin, on the other hand, is pure protein but lacks the essential amino acid tryptophan. A number of plant foods are deficient in one or more of the essential amino acids. All cereal grains are deficient in lysine; rice and corn are also lacking threonine and tryptophan. Peas, beans, and other lequmes are deficient in methionine and tryptophan. Soybeans and seed oils are low in methionine. By combining different foods with complimentary amino acids it may be possible to obtain a satisfactory amino acid balance. Because of the necessary reactions between amino acids and their dependence upon each other for these reactions, a diet containing only a small amount of one essential amino acid will reduce the available amino acids in the rest of the diet. All amino acids must be present at the same time before they can be utilized as protein. In other words, the chain is only as strong as its weakest link. The excess amino acids that can not be used as protein because of insufficient complimentary amino acids are used as energy or excreted. Amino acids cannot be stored for future use as protein.

Amino acids are broken down and released in the intestinal tract during ingestion of food protein and are carried by the blood stream to the body cells where they are used for growth, repair, muscles, red blood cells, body tissue, and general maintenance. During cellular anabolism (buildup) amino acids join together by peptide bonds to form specific proteins. With cellular catabolism (breakdown), proteins and amino acid chains are broken up into fragments.

Note: Amino acids are classified as either D (d): dextrorotational, which means they bend polarized light (light through a prism) to the right, or L (l): levorotational, which means they bend polarized light to the left. The L classification of amino acids are the group generally ingested.

Use for MENTAL ASSIST & to CORRECT A DEFICIENCY

Practitioners and Researchers: at www.LifeEnergyResearch.com, complete the SAF-120 Questionnaire, then access your account at SAFonline and use the Amino Acid Interpretation to determine which amino acids are best for the client based on that chain.

The Self Awareness Formulas (SAF®) employ homeopathic amino acids as a mental assist technique (not for physical correction of symptomatology). As noted previously, amino acids are the building blocks of protein. The DNA in the protein structures of organs and glands contain all the information of the traumas and lifetime events. For SAF emotional release work, we use amino acids to assist the client in clarifying mental images.

Homeopathy, from the Greek, "homeos" (meaning similar) and "pathos" (suffering), has risen in popularity because it espouses natural laws of healing and uses herbs, minerals, and other substances to achieve this end. Joe Scogna, the founder of SAF®, defined homeopathic products as "light polarizers" in that they expand energy. When used in SAF chain work to clarify the content of mental images, the dose is 3 to 5 drops under the tongue, every 5 to 10 minutes, for at least an hour or until the image is located. Then the product is discontinued. Again, with this type of emotional release work, no attempt is made to correct symptomatology.

Those who practice homeopathy follow the premise that the body needs only minute doses to bring about change. Homeopathic products are potentized, or highly diluted. If the ingredient is listed as "6x" this means there is one part substance to 1,000,000 parts distilled water. This potentized dilution contains the electrical energy of the original substance; these light polarizers stimulate and realign energies into various positions that are easier for the body to handle on an energetic level.

The following list of antidotes should be avoided when taking any homeopathic dilutions:
    All mints (snacks, cosmetics, toothpaste, teas)
    Camphor (menthol, eucalyptus)
    Pain killers (aspirin, etc), narcotic drugs, OTC products
    Analgesic rubs (Ben Gay)
    Stimulants/caffeine (coffee, tea, tonic water, soda)

The Amino Acid Interpretation through SAFonline can also be used by practitioners for finding deficiencies. Complete the SAF-120 Questionnaire and run the chain through the Amino Acid Interpretation to find what amino acids will provide balance.

Theoretically, we should be able to get all the amino acids from the foods we eat, but because of eating habits and the complex stresses of our modern life most practitioners agree supplementation is necessary.

Deficiencies occur in several ways. Low-protein and vegetarian diets, where the proper combining of vegetable proteins is skipped, can result in lowered levels of arginine, glutamine, glycine, taurine and other amino acids.

Fatty, rich foods that produce an excess of uric acid in the system can lead to gout AND low levels of alanine, aspartic acid, glutamic acid and glycine. Because the liver is the site where amino acids are metabolized, those with damaged livers, such as from drug use and especially alcoholics, have abnormally low levels of isoleucine, leucine and valine.

Chronic exposure to toxins (chemicals in the food, polluted air, and city water) also cause depletion of the above amino acids, as well as low levels of methionine and cysteine.

People who exercise, especially weight lifters, need extra protein and amino acids to help replace lost protein and to build up muscle mass.

Practitioners have reported that supplements of the amino acids alanine, glutamic acid and glycine have controlled the symptoms of an enlarged prostate gland in men. Tryptophan, which raises the serotonin level in the brain, has been used to relieve depression and aid in sleep disorders.

Practitioners who recommend amino acids for their clients often suggest supplements in gel cap or pill form. These are processed products. In late 1989, the entire USA supply of tryptophan, imported through a Japanese company, was found to be "tainted". Look for products that state on the bottle: "contains only naturally occurring L-tryptophan."

This book, *Amino Acids—a Nutritional Guide*, can be utilized for both mental assists and for deficiencies:, access the Interpretation through www.LifeEnergyResearch.com/SAFonline.

 —Essential Amino Acids, those that must be supplied by foods or outside sources, are designated on the following pages by a star. See also List, page 45.

Alanine

Alanine was discovered in protein in 1875. It is not essential to the human diet as it can be made in the body from other metabolites. Its side chain participates in hydrophobic interactions.

$$H_2N - \underset{H}{\overset{CH_3}{\underset{|}{\overset{|}{C}}}} - C\underset{OH}{\overset{O}{\diagup}}$$

Alanine

Suggested nutritional use:
    burn out
    convulsions
    improper diet
    electric surge (nerves)
    mental deterioration
    spastic movements
    hyper-muscular contractions
    insufficient rest
    sweats at night
    tic
    twitches

Glands Affected:
    thymus
    hypothalamus
    eye
    pineal
    thyroid
    brain

Complementary Vitamins:
- C***
- A*
- niacin*
- B-complex*
- B12
- B3
- B15
- E
- B2
- PABA
- pantothenic acid

Complementary Minerals:
- chromium
- zinc
- calcium
- selenium
- magnesium
- sulfur

Arginine ☆

Arginine was discovered in protein in 1895. It is usually considered essential for children as it is necessary for the maintenance of normal growth rate. Arginine is a direct precursor of urea, the dominant nitrogenous waste product of most mammals. It is used intravenously as an adjunct in the management of excess ammonia in the blood.

$$H_2C - NH - C - NH_2$$
$$| \quad\quad\quad ||$$
$$CH_2 \quad\quad NH$$
$$|$$
$$CH_2$$
$$|\quad\quad\quad O$$
$$H_2N - C - C$$
$$|\quad\quad\quad OH$$
$$H$$

Arginine

Suggested nutritional use:
- proper growth in children
- growth hormone releaser
- wound healer
- weight control
- immune system stimulant
- for fat loss
- muscle increase
- arthritis
- detoxification of poisonous wastes
- sterility (comprises 80% of seminal fluid)
- intestinal problems
- cellulite
- non-specific infection or inflammation
- pelvic stress
- calcification
- inflamed veins
- deficiency of vitamin B6

Glands Affected:
- hypothalamus
- eye
- pineal
- thymus
- lymph
- tonsils
- appendix
- pyres patches
- skin
- parathyroid

Complementary Vitamins:
- A**
- niacin
- C
- B-complex
- B15
- E

Complementary Minerals:
- calcium
- selenium
- magnesium
- sulfur

Aspartic Acid

Aspartic acid was discovered in protein in 1868. It is not essential to the diet. Its acidic side chain (negative charge) offers more water solublity to protein and it is involved with some enzyme activity (pepsin).

Aspartic acid

Suggested nutritional use:
    gall bladder dysfunction
    liver troubles

Glands Affected:
    pancreas
    solar plexus
    spine
    liver
    stomach
    spleen
    thymus

Complementary Vitamins:
    B-complex**
    A*
    pantothenic acid
    B_6
    niacin
    choline
    inositol
    B_2
    B_{12}

folic acid
C

Complementary Minerals:
  chromium
  zinc
  lead
  gold
  iron
  nickel
  manganese
  copper
  potassium
  bromine
  sodium
  chloride

Asparagine

Asparagine was the first amino acid isolated from a natural source, asparagus juice, in 1806, but it was not until 1932 that proof of the occurance of this amino acid in protein was found. It is not essential to the diet as the human body can synthesize it from aspartic acid. Its chemical structure is identical to that of aspartic acid except one side chain is linked to ammonia making it an amide. Asparagine is necessary for the metabolism of toxic ammonia in the body.

$$H_2N-\underset{\underset{H}{|}}{\overset{\overset{\displaystyle C(=O)NH_2}{|}}{\underset{}{C}}}-C(=O)OH \quad \text{with } CH_2 \text{ linker}$$

Asparagine

Suggested nutritional use:
    gall bladder dysfunction
    liver troubles

Glands Affected:
    lymph
    thymus
    liver

Complementary Vitamins:
    A*
    niacin
    choline
    inositol

Complementary Minerals:
    chromium
    zinc

Cysteine and Cystine

Cystine was isolated from a urinary calculi in 1810 and from horn tissue in 1899. The reduction of cystine to cysteine was reported in 1884 and the chemical structures of the two amino acids were made by chemical synthesis in 1903-1904. Two cysteine molecules linked together create cystine. Neither cysteine or cystine are essential to the diet of man; cystine and cysteine are interconfertable and cysteine is created in the body from serine and methionine. It is particularly abundant in the protein of hair, hooves and keratin of the skin. A hair "permanent" works by breaking, rearranging and re-forming disulphide bridges of hair protein. It participates in the catalytic reaction of certain enzymes such as papain in meat tenderizers. Chains of cysteine link up to form insulin and it is needed for proper structure of proteins and enzymes.

Cystinuria, an inherited metabolic disease, has as one of its symptoms, a twenty to thirty-fold increase in urinary excretion of cystine, impairing kidney function. Another inherited disease, cystinosis, causes renal failure.

Cysteine

Cystine

Suggested nutritional use:
> cigarette smokers
> aging
> drinkers
> arthritis
> hair and skin
> astigmatism
> blurred images
> eye troubles
> myopic eyes
> gout
> migraine headache
> rheumatism
> systemic poison; deposits in joints
> systemic poison: flows

Glands Affected:
> adrenal

Complementary Vitamins:
> pantothenic acid
> C

Complementary Minerals:
> potassium
> sodium

Glutamic Acid

This amino acid was isolated from wheat gluten in 1866 and chemically made in 1890. It is not an essential amino acid.

Glutamic acid serves as an acceptor and donor of ammonia. When coupled with ammonia, it becomes glutamine and can safely transport ammonia to the liver where it becomes urea and is excreted by the kidneys. Glutamic acid can also be converted and degraded to carbon dioxide and water and transformed into sugar for the Krebs Cycle of energy. Glutamic acid increases the water solubility of a protein. Monosodium glutamate (MSG) is widely used as a condiment.

Glutamic acid

Suggested nutritional use:
- brain upsets
- mood swings
- brown out
- slow death
- detrimental diet
- loss of energy ignition
- malnutrition
- increased urination
- wasting water

Glands Affected:
- adrenal
- pancreas
- solar plexus
- spine

Complementary Vitamins:
- pantothenic acid*
- C
- B-complex
- B6
- niacin

Complementary Minerals:
- potassium
- sodium
- chromium
- zinc

Glutamine

Glutamine was isolated from beet juice in 1883 but not isolated from a protein until 1932. It was chemically synthesized in 1933. It is a non-essential amino acid as it can be made in the body from glutamic acid. Its chemical structure is identical to glutamic acid except for the addition of ammonia, creating an amide. The glutamic acid-glutamine interaction is of central importance to the regulation of the toxic levels of ammonia in the body. When amino acid concentrations are evaluated in blood plasma, glutamine is highest. Glutamine participates in creating urea (for excretion by the kidneys) and purines (genetic DNA material).

Glutamine

Suggested nutritional use:
    breathing difficulties caused by heart troubles
    flu
    cardiac dyspnea

Glands Affected:
    lymph
    thymus
    heart

Complimentary Vitamins:
    A
    niacin
    E

Complimentary Minerals:
    chromium
    zinc
    calcium
    selenium
    magnesium
    sulfur

Glycine

Glycine was the first amino acid to be isolated from protein gelatin. It is not essential to the diet as the body can make it from other substances. It is structurally the simplest of the amino acids. Glycine is needed for biosynthesis of heme (component of hemoglobin) and biosynthesis of serine, purines (DNA) and gluthathione (co-enzymes). It is an inhibitory neuro-transmitter in the central nervous system.

$$H_2N-\underset{H}{\overset{H}{C}}-C\underset{OH}{\overset{O}{\diagup}}$$

Glycine

Suggested nutritional use:

    disturbed oxygen-carbon dioxide balance
    heart trouble
    difficult or labored breathing
    cardio/pulmonary disturbance
    decreased activity of neurons

Glands Affected:

    thyroid*
    bone
    heart
    liver
    spleen

Complementary Vitamins:

    C**
    A*
    E*
    niacin
    B_2

PABA
B-complex

Complementary Minerals:
magnesium
sulfur

Histidine ⭐

Histidine was isolated from protein in 1896 and its chemical structure was confirmed in 1911. Histidine must be supplied in the diet of children; experiments indicate adults can go for only short periods of time without this amino acid. Histidine is a direct precursor of histamine, one of the healing type chemicals released from cells upon tissue injury or in neutralization of antigens. It is also an important source of carbon atoms in the creation of purines (genetic material, DNA). Histidine can act as an acid and as a base - it can donate and accept protons, works with enzymes and participates in the function of chymotrypsin as well as the metabolism of carbohydrates, proteins, and nucleic acids.

Histidine (structural diagram)

Suggested nutritional use:
- proper growth of children
- hallucinations
- paranoia
- deafness
- hard of hearing
- proper functioning of auditory nerves
- enhances sexual orgasm
- chelates copper and zinc
- impotence
- arthritis
- bowel dysfunction

aids digestion
reduced flow of creativity
electric flow reduced
pineal disturbances
male-reduced flow of semen
loss of vigor
loss of sexual power

Glands Affected:
adrenal

Complementary Vitamins:
pantothenic acid*
C
niacin
E

Complementary Minerals:
potassium
bromine
sodium
chloride
chromium
zinc

Hydroxyproline

In 1902, hydroxyproline was isolated from gelatin. It was synthesized during the years 1905-1919. It is present in collagen-connective tissue, skin, ligaments, tendons, bone and cartilage.

Hydroxyproline

Suggested nutritional use:
    decaying of bones
    dizziness
    electric charge in spine is uncoordinated
    hyperthyroid
    nerves overtaxed
    deficiency of vitamin D
    rickets
    sciatica
    gradual deterioration of the spine
    decaying of teeth
    thigh pain
    gradual hardening and loss of function of vital organs

Glands Affected:
    thyroid
    parathyroid

Complementary Vitamins:
    C
    niacin
    B2

PABA
A

Complementary Minerals:
 lithium
 fluorine
 sodium
 chloride
 calcium
 selenium
 magnesium
 sulfur

Isoleucine ⭐

Isoleucine was isolated from beet sugar molasses in 1904. It is an essential amino acid. Young adults need about 20 mg per day per kilogram of body weight. In rare inherited cases, imbalances of isoleucine, leucine and valine can cause a buildup of certain metabolites in the urine creating the disease called Maple Sugar Urine Disease. Isoleucine participates in hydrophobic interactions.

$$H_2N-\underset{\underset{H}{|}}{\overset{\overset{CH_3}{|}}{\underset{|}{\overset{|}{C}}}}\underset{}{\overset{CHCH_3}{|}} - C\overset{O}{\underset{OH}{\diagup\diagdown}}$$

Isoleucine

Suggested nutritional use:
    hemoglobin formation
    flu
    gravel in the urine
    hemoglobin in the urine

Glands Affected:
    thymus*
    lymph
    hypothalamus
    eye
    pineal
    kidney

Complementary Vitamins:
   A***
   niacin*
   C*
   B-complex
   B15
   E
   B12

Complementary Minerals:
   chromium
   zinc
   calcium
   selenium
   magnesium
   sulfur

Leucine ⭐

Leucine was isolated from cheese in 1819 and from muscle and wool in 1820. Because when purified it was a white crystalline substance, the compound was named Leucine after the Greek word Leukos, meaning white. The structure of leucine was synthesized in 1891. It is an essential amino acid-young adults need about 31 mg daily of this amino acid per kilogram of body weight.

$$\begin{array}{c} CH_3 \quad CH_3 \\ \diagdown \; \diagup \\ CH \\ | \\ CH_2 \\ | \\ H_2N - C - C\diagup^O \\ | \quad\quad \diagdown OH \\ H \end{array}$$

Leucine

Suggested nutritional use:
- inability to gain or lose weight
- digestive problems
- colon spasms
- stress
- problems of civilized man
- congested liver
- kidney damage

Glands Affected:
- thymus
- lymph
- tonsils
- appendix
- pyres patches
- skin
- stomach

Complementary Vitamins:
- A
- B-complex
- B2
- B12
- folic acid

Complementary Minerals:
- **copper**
- **manganese**
- **calcium**
- **selenium**

Lysine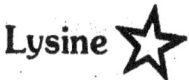

Lysine was first isolated from casein (milk protein) in 1889 and laboratory synthesis was complete in 1902. Lysine is an essential amino acid; young adults need 23 mg per day per kilogram of body weight. Lysine is found in very low concentrations in cereal proteins. Wheat gluten is particularly a poor source. Proper growth of children and general well being of adults fails in diets depending on cereal proteins as a sole source of essential amino acids. Lysine is necessary for binding the co-enzymes pyridoxal phosphate, lipoic acid, and biotin with enzymes.

Lysine

Suggested nutritional use for:
    antibody formation
    chronic tiredness
    fatigue
    red lines in the eyes
    nausea
    dizziness
    anemia
    formation of glutamic acid
    depression
    diminishing control
    loss of/ill effects of companion, ally or loved one
    buildup of environmental pressures
    helplessness

homesickness
destruction of electric current carrying fibers
hypoglycemia
mental trouble
losing muscular integrity

Glands Affected:

pancreas
solar plexus
spine
hypothalamus
eye
pineal
thyroid
brain
adrenal

Complementary Vitamins:

niacin***
B-complex**
C**
pantothenic acid*
B6
A
B15
E
B2
PABA

Complementary Minerals:

chromium
zinc
rubidium
iodine
sodium
chloride

Methionine ⭐

Methionine was found in casein (milk protein) in 1922 and synthesized in the laboratory in 1928. It is an essential amino acid. Thirty-one mg per day per body weight must be supplied by the diet. Methionine contributes to the synthesis of epinephrine (the hormone adrenelin) and choline (the essential part of lecithin and acetcholine, the neuro transmitter). Adrenalin is a heart stimulant, vasoconstrictor, useful to lower intra-occular pressure in glaucoma treatment.

$$H_2N-\underset{H}{\overset{CH_2-CH_2-SCH_3}{C}}-C\underset{OH}{\overset{O}{\diagup\diagdown}}$$

Methionine

Suggested nutritional use:
- anti-oxidant
- low blood sugar
- cardio-vascular disease
- bowel dysfunction
- emotional drainers surround the individual
- energy thief in the vicinity
- intestinal problems
- heavy metal action
- hypoglycemia
- kidney and liver cells
- stimulates hair growth
- helps eliminate toxic waste from the body
- relieves rheumatic aches and pains
- furnishes sulfur for formation of cysteine/cystine

Glands Affected:
 thymus*
 lymph
 adrenal

Complementary Vitamins:
 A*
 C*
 niacin
 B12
 pantothenic acid

Complementary Minerals:
 chromium
 zinc

Phenylalanine ⭐

Phenylalanine was isolated from lupine sprouts in 1879 and chemically synthesized in 1882. It is an essential amino acid. Young adults need 31 mg per day kilogram of body weight. Enzymes degrade phenylalanine into simpler compounds and also convert it to the amino acid tyrosine. Failure of the enzymes to make this conversion results in phenylketonuria, or too much phenylalanine in the blood which causes mental retardation. A PKU test to determine this is performed a couple of days after birth, if diagnosed early enough PKU can be controlled by a diet very low in phenylalanine. This amino acid participates in hydrophobic interactions.

Phenylalanine

Suggested nutritional use:
- depression
- growth hormone stimulant
- mood elevator
- longer attention span
- weight control
- appetite blocker
- body defense forces in retreat
- more forthright in personality
- swollen glands
- disturbed anal area
- rectal calculi

tumor arising from a serous or mucous surface
proper metabolism
thyroid troubles
blood vessels
sparks nerve activity
mental balance

Glands Affected:
parathyroid
hypothalamus
eye
pineal

Complementary Vitamins:
A*
niacin
C
B-complex
B_{15}
E

Complementary Minerals:
calcium
selenium
magnesium
sulfur

Proline

In 1900, Proline's chemical synthesis occured even before its isolation from a natural source. In 1901, the natural structure was found in casein (milk protein).

It is not essential to the human diet because it can be created in the body from glutamic acid. Because of the nature of its chemical structure, proline figures prominently in the shape or type of protein created. Collagen, the fibrous protein of connective tissue, is comprised of 21% proline.

Proline

Suggested nutritional use:

    cardiac dysfunction
    heart trouble
    skin problems

Glands Affected:

    bone
    duodenum
    stomach
    heart
    liver
    spleen
    thyroid

Complementary Vitamins:

    A**
    E**

B-complex*
C*
niacin
trypsin
chymotrypsin
B2
B12
folic acid

Complementary Minerals:
    magnesium
    sulfur
    aluminum
    phosphorus
    calcium
    selenium
    chromium;
    zinc

Serine

In 1865, Serine was first obtained from silk protein and its structure was synthesized in 1902. It can be synthesized in the body from other metabolites such as glycine so it is not essential to the diet. Serine is very important in metabolism. It plays an important role in the catalytic function of enzymes. The nerve gases and insecticides work by combining with a residue of serine which then inhibits proper enzyme activity and the neurotransmitter acetycholine reaches dangerous high levels quickly, resulting in convulsions and death.

$$H_2N-\underset{H}{\overset{CH_2OH}{C}}-C\overset{O}{\underset{OH}{\diagup\!\!\!\!\diagdown}}$$

Serine

Suggested nutritional use:
  common cough
  electric hypermotion
  hypersensing
  nervousness

Glands Affected:
  brain
  stomach
  pancreas
  solar plexus
  spine
  hypothalamus
  eye
  pineal

Complementary Vitamins:
  B-complex***
  C

pantothenic acid*
niacin*
B2
B12
folic acid
B6
A
B15
E

Complementary Minerals:
calcium
selenium
magnesium
sulfur
chromium
zinc

Threonine ⭐

Threonine was first isolated from the protein fibrin in 1935 and synthesized in the lab later that same year. Threonine is an essential amino acid; young adults need 14 mg per day per kilogram of body weight. This amino acid participates in biosynthesis of vitamin B12 and isoleucine. It is useful in many reactions of bacteria.

$$H_2N - \underset{H}{\underset{|}{C}} - \overset{\overset{CH_3}{|}}{\underset{|}{C}}HOH - C\overset{O}{\underset{OH}{\diagup}}$$

Threonine

Suggested nutritional use:

    indigestion
    intestinal malfunctions
    liver fat
    lack of defense against colds
    female-ovarian cysts/fluid on ovary(s)
    diminishing defense against infection or flu
    female-dysmenorrhea/menstruation   painful/difficult/
        spotting/intermittent
    inflamed uterus

Glands Affected:

    thymus
    lymph
    tonsils
    appendix
    pyres patches
    skin
    stomach

Complementary Vitamins:
- A
- B-complex
- B_2
- B_{12}
- folic acid

Complementary Minerals:
- copper
- manganese
- calcium
- selenium

Tryptophan ⭐

First isolated from casein (milk protein) in 1901, tryptophan's structure was established in 1907. It is essential to the human diet and cannot be synthesized from other sources. Young adults need about 7 mg per day per kilogram of body weight. Nicotinic acid (niacin or vitamin B3) can be made from tryptophan in the body but the process is too slow and inadequate for normal growth and development and thus nicotinic acid must be supplied in the diet. Pellegra, a vitamin deficiency disease, is made worse by a diet low in tryptophan. Intestinal bacteria break tryptophan down into the compounds indole and skatole, which are mainly responsible for the unpleasant odor of feces. Tryptophan participates in hydrophobic interactions. It is essential for optimum growth in infants and for nitrogen equilibrium in adults. Tryptophan helps bring on sleep; narcoleptics seem abnormally sensitive to this amino acid causing uncontrollable sleep. Adequate levels in the diet may compensate for deficiencies of niacin and thus mitigate pellagra. Sixty mg of tryptophan can substitute for one mg of niacin.

Tryptophan

Suggested nutritional use:

    aids in prevention of pellegra
    raise blood histimine
    B6 deficiency
    flu
    proper brain metabolism
    skin and hair
    nerves

schizophrenia
increases muscle strength
wakefulness at night
lower blood cholesterol
dermatitis on dorsal surface of hands and back of neck
aids utilization of B-complex group especially B6
alcoholism
relieves migraine headaches
growth hormone stimulant
arthritis
digestive aid
joint dysfunctions

Glands Affected:

parathyroid
lymph
thymus
lung
spleen

Complementary Vitamins:

A**
niacin
E

Complementary Minerals:

calcium
selenium
magnesium
sulfur

Tyrosine

Tyrosine was obtained from cheese in 1846 and in 1883 its structure was synthesized in the laboratory. It can be created in the body by phenylalanine so it is not considered an essential amino acid. When the enzyme which activates the conversion of phenylalanine to tyrosine is not active because of a defect, Phenylketonuria (PKU) results and can lead to mental retardation if not treated quickly. Another disorder caused by upsets of tyrosine metabolism is alkaptonuria (urine which darkens upon exposure to air). Tyrosine is a precursor to the adrenal hormones ephin- ephrin and norepinephrin and the thyroid hormones thyroxin and melanine (skin and hair pigments).

Tyrosine

Suggested nutritional use
    anti-depressant
    affects blood pressure (can lower or raise)
    protects against free radicals by bonding (don't take if
       already have melanoma)
    for weight loss
    appetite inhibitor
    muscle growth
    anti-oxidant
    anti-aging

atrophy
reduced flow of creativity
electric flow reduced
impotence
pineal disturbances
male-reduced flow of semen
loss of vigor

Glands Affected:

anterior pituitary
thymus
lymph
tonsils
appendix
adrenal
pyres patches
skin

Complementary Vitamins:

A*
C*
E
pantothenic acid

Complementary Minerals:

calcium
selenium
magnesium

Valine ☆

Valine was first isolated from albumin in 1879 and its structure was established in 1906. It is essential to the human diet. Young adults need about 23 mg per day per kilogram of body weight. An inherited defect in one of the enzymes derived from valine results in Maple Sugar Urine Disease. Valine participates in hydrophobic interactions.

$$H_2N-\underset{\underset{H}{|}}{\overset{\overset{\displaystyle CH(CH_3)_2}{|}}{C}}-C\underset{OH}{\overset{O}{\diagup\!\!\!\diagdown}}$$

Valine

Suggested nutritional use:

    spitting up blood
    cell deterioration
    viral invasion of chest cavity
    erythema
    abnormal reddening of skin
    tension
    inflammation of the lower part of the throat
    laser stimulated reaction
    rectum inflamed
    muscles
    mental and emotional upsets
    insomnia
    nervousness

Glands Affected:

    thymus
    lymph
    tonsils

appendix
pyres patches
skin
duodenum
heart
liver
spleen
thyroid
posterior pituitary

Complementary Vitamins:

A***
C*
E*
trypsin
chymotrypsin
niacin
B-complex

Complementary Minerals:

copper
manganese
magnesium
sulfur

Essential Amino Acids

Amino acids are considered essential if they cannot be produced by the body processes or created by combinations of other amino acids. Essential amino acids must be supplied by diet for proper functioning of body and mind.

- Arginine
- Histidine
- Isoleucine
- Leucine
- Lysine
- Methionine
- Phenylalanine
- Threonine
- Tryptophan
- Valine

References

Amino Acids—a Nutritional Guide
    Kathy M. Scogna, 1983, 2005
Amino Acid Fractionization
    Bio Center Laboratory 1980
Amino Acid Sorter (SAF QUIRK file)
    Joseph R. Scogna, Jr. 1983
Amino-22 Database (Mapscribe) Life Energy System
    Joseph R. Scogna, Jr. 1983
Basic Monitor Course Series
    Joseph R. Scogna, Jr. 1988
Dorland's Illustrated Medical Dictionary
    William B. Saunders, Inc. 1974
Life Extension
    Durk Pearson and Sandy Shaw 1982
Mental and Elemental Nutrients
    Dr. Carl Pfeiffer 1975
Merck Manual
    Merck and Co, Inc 1977

Index

Adrenal hormones, 29, 41
Alanine, 5
Alcoholics, 4
Amino acid interpretation, 3, 4
Amino acids, contents of, 1
Ammonia, toxic levels, 7, 11, 14, 16
Antidotes of homeopathic, 4
Arginine, 7
Asparagine, 11
Asparagus juice, 11
Aspartic acid, 9

Building blocks of protein, 1

Cereal, poor source, 27
Co-enzymes, 18, 27
Collagen, 22, 33
Customized work-ups, inside back cover
Cysteine, 12
Cystine, 12
Cystinuria, 12

D classification of, 2
Deficiencies of, 4

Energy thief, 29
Enzymes, 7, 12, 20
Essential amino acids, 1, 4, 45 (list)
Essential to plant and animal life, 1
Exercise and depletion, 4
Exposure to toxins, 4

Fatty foods and effects, 4

Glutamic acid, 14
Glutamine, 16
Glycine, 18
Growth rate, 7

Hair permanent, 12
Heme, biosynthesis of, 18
Histamine precursor, 20
Histidine, 20
Homeopathic amino acids, 3
Homeopathic dilutions, 3
Hydroxyproline, 22

Increase serotonin levels, 4
Insecticides, 35
Insulin, 12
Introduction, 1
Isoleucine, 24

Joe Scogna, 3

L classification of, 2
Leucine, 26
Light polarizers, 3
Lysine, 27

Maple sugar urine disease, 24, 43
Mental assist technique, 3
Methionine, 29
MSG, 16

Neuro-transmitter, 18, 29, 35
Niacin deficiency, 39

Pellegra, 39
Pepsin, 9
Phenylalanine, 31
PKU, 31, 41
Plants deficient, 2
Polarized light, bend, 2
Proline, 33
Protein of hair, skin, 12
Protoplasm, 1

SAF use of amino acids, 3
SAFonline, 3, 4, inside back cover
Serine, 35
Sleep aid, 39

Threonine, 37
Thyroid hormones, 41
Tryptophan, 39
    supply tainted, 4
Tyrosine, 41

Use for mental assist, 3

Valine, 43
Vegetarian diets, 4

Wakefulness at night, 40

Create customized Work-ups with SAF Online!

Go to www.LifeEnergyResearch.com

1. Click on SAFonline, open an account (email address and password) for the time period you desire. Pay as you go or economical yearly rates.
2. Create a file for you, taking note of your Client KEY.
3. Click on "Questionnaire" (three are available at no charge) Choose one, enter a complaint, something that you want to work on; something that is stopping or hindering you.
4. Complete the Questionnaire, receive your chain of numbers, and enter your client KEY. Once you click Submit, all chain data will go automatically into the file you created. Read about your numbers in *SAF Simplified* or *The Numbers of SAF*.
5. Follow the directions on the screen. Click on chain, and choose the Amino Acids Interpretation to find what amino acids mat assist with balance. Refer to this book for history, complementary vitamins, minerals and synergists.
6. At SAF Online, you'll find MANY other exciting Interpretations to invigorate your practice and research work. (Herbs, Antigens, Essential oils, Flower Essences, Homeopathic Remedies, Business Solutions, Colors, Acupuncture Points, Chinese Herbs and many more!

No two people are the same;
with SAF, no two solutions will ever be the same either!

 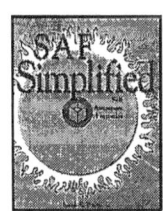 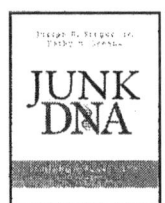 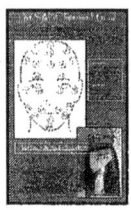

Learn more about the Self Awareness Formulas (SAF®)

Read: The Numbers of SAF; SAF Simplified; Junk DNA; SAF Infrared Manual

SAF Road Map, Level 1 Training: theory and practical. 5 books; 5 hours personal work with SAF practitioner, free weeks of SAF online service. $690

www.ingramcontent.com/pod-product-compliance
Lightning Source LLC
Chambersburg PA
CBHW071823170526
45167CB00003B/1399